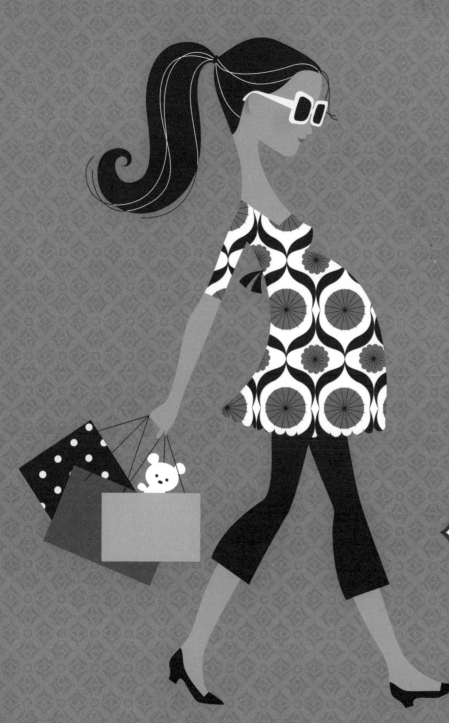

# My Pregnancy

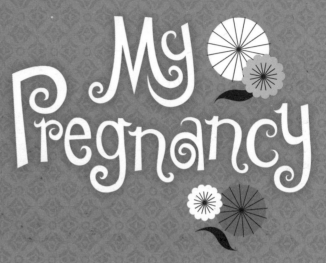

The day I started this journal:

_____

new seasons®

To
Our beautiful daughter Amy,
We are so excited for you
and love you so much!
♡ All our love ♡
M & D

**Stacy Peterson** ®

Artwork © Stacy Peterson®
All rights reserved.
www.stacypeterson.net

New Seasons is a registered trademark of Publications International, Ltd.

Louis Weber, CEO
Publications International, Ltd.
8140 Lehigh Avenue
Morton Grove, Illinois 60053

**www.pilbooks.com**

ISBN-13: 978-1-4508-6202-8
ISBN-10: 1-4508-6202-0

Manufactured in China.

8 7 6 5 4 3 2 1

# Contents

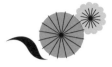
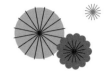

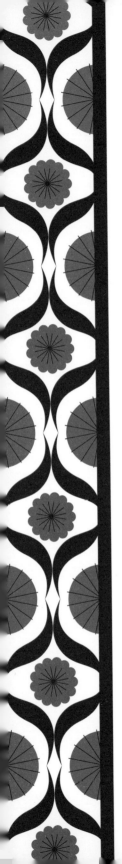

# Welcome to Your Pregnancy Journal

Congratulations, you are now entering the wonderful, topsy-turvy world of motherhood! This is one of the most important times of your life as well as the most complex and memorable. This journal is dedicated to you and all of the up-and-down moments of your pregnancy. You can easily record special, momentous, and comical events, as you experience them, in each trimester. There are also checklists and design pages to help you plan for your little one's arrival. Once baby is born, you will enjoy reliving the honest, heartwarming moments you have captured in this book. When your child is older, he or she will also appreciate being able to look back over such an exciting time.

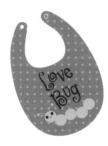

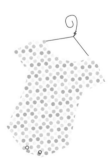

Is not a young mother one of the sweetest sights life shows us?

— William Makepeace Thackeray

# A Wish Come True!

The day I met your daddy... _____

_____

_____

I knew I wanted to start a family with him because... _____

_____

_____

I first suspected I was pregnant when... _____

_____

Place a profile photo of you at the very beginning of your pregnancy here.

Thoughts: _____

_____

_____

_____

_____

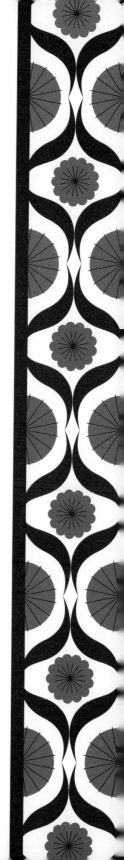

# Surprise, Surprise!

How I decided to tell your daddy… _____

_____

_____

_____

_____

His reaction… _____

_____

_____

_____

_____

_____

_____

_____

_____

# Sharing the News!

We planned to wait until _____ to tell everyone the news.

Who we told first… _____

_____

_____

_____

Some of the best reactions… _____

_____

_____

_____

_____

We celebrated by… _____

_____

_____

_____

# My First Prenatal Visit

My wonderful doctor: _____

My expected due date: _____

My first ultrasound was on _____ and took place at _____

_____

The people who went to this appointment with me… _____

_____

The first thing I saw on the ultrasound screen… _____

_____

_____

I felt… _____

_____

_____

Everyone else in the room said… _____

_____

Important information I received from my doctor/technician… _____

_____

# Baby's First Picture

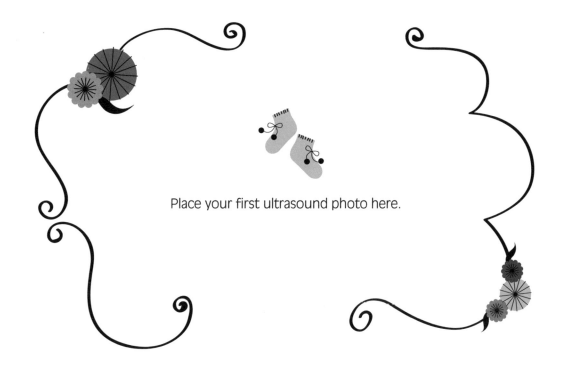

Place your first ultrasound photo here.

Thoughts: _____

_____

_____

_____

_____

# Heartbeats of Love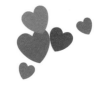

Date and time of the appointment: _____

The first time I heard your heartbeat… _____

_____

_____

_____

The doctor said… _____

_____

_____

_____

Your daddy said he felt… _____

_____

_____

_____

After leaving the doctor's office that day... _____

_____

_____

_____

_____

_____

_____

_____

_____

_____

_____

_____

_____

_____

_____

_____

_____

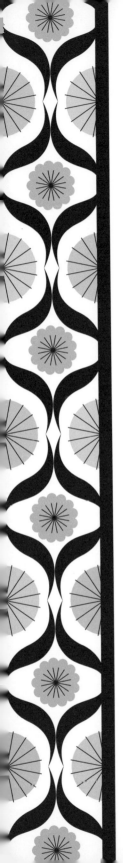

# Nibble & Nosh

During the first trimester, my appetite has been (check all that apply):

____ nonexistent          ____ voracious          ____ the same

____ increasing by the day          ____ other: _____

The foods I can't get by without… _____

_____

_____

Smells that make me queasy… _____

_____

_____

My weirdest cravings… _____

_____

_____

My biggest helpers in the kitchen… _____

_____

_____

# A New Routine

I started these new habits when I knew you were on the way… _____

_____

_____

_____

My new exercise program includes… _____

_____

_____

_____

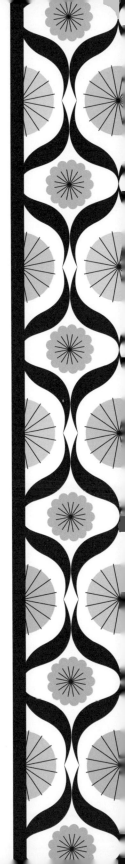

Some hobbies that I enjoy…_____

_____

_____

How Daddy and I spend our weekends now… _____

_____

_____

A fun getaway… _____

_____

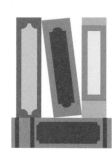

# Favorite Pregnancy Reads

List some favorite books, articles, or websites you've read while you're expecting.

Title: _____

Author:_____

Title: _____

Author: _____

Title: _____

Author: _____

Websites:_____

_____

_____

The most important things I've learned… _____

_____

_____

_____

_____

# Summing It Up

**During the first trimester...**

My emotions have been... _____

_____

_____

_____

_____

My symptoms (the good, the bad, and the moody)... _____

_____

_____

_____

_____

Some noteworthy events... _____

_____

_____

_____

Date _____

**Reflections on my first trimester...**

_____

_____

_____

_____

_____

_____

_____

_____

_____

_____

_____

_____

_____

Date _____

# The Second Trimester

**The day my belly really popped:** _____ / _____ / _____

How I felt about it… _____

_____

_____

_____

Now I need to… _____

_____

_____

_____

Other people's reactions to my bump… _____

_____

_____

_____

# Snapshot

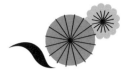
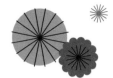

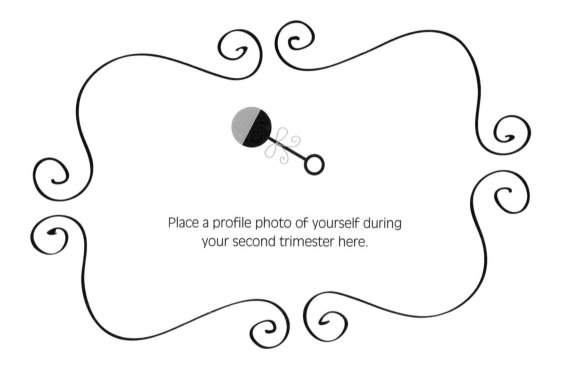

Place a profile photo of yourself during your second trimester here.

Thoughts: _____

_____

_____

_____

_____

# Mommy Chic

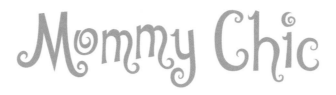

I first started buying maternity clothes… _____

_____

_____

_____

It was a relief because… _____

_____

_____

_____

I'm going to miss wearing… _____

_____

_____

_____

Pregnancy fashion tips and tricks I've learned… _____

_____

_____

_____

My favorite maternity outfits… _____

_____

_____

_____

Clothes I borrowed from my friends… _____

_____

_____

_____

The staple pieces I've worn again and again… _____

_____

_____

Outfits for special events… _____

_____

_____

_____

If I could design maternity clothes, this is what I would change… _____

_____

_____

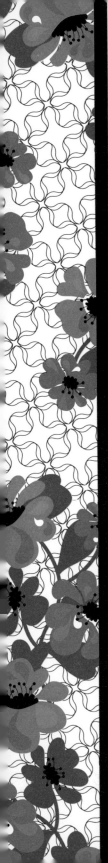

# Haute Mama

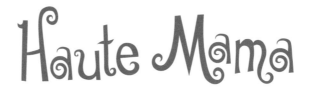

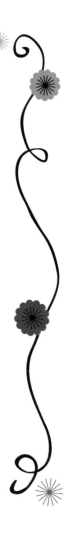

Place a photo of you in your
favorite maternity ensemble here.

Thoughts: _____

_____

_____

_____

_____

# Pretty 'n' Pampered

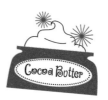

Cocoa Butter

I unwind at the end of the day by… _____

_____

_____

_____

My favorite places to relax… _____

_____

_____

_____

Since being pregnant, I've treated myself to… _____

_____

_____

_____

My friends and family spoil me by… _____

_____

_____

_____

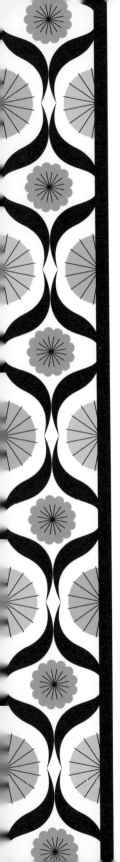

# The Gender Reveal

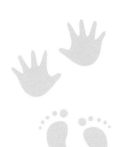

**We've made up our minds to (check one):**

_____ find out!                    _____ wait until you arrive!

Why we decided to… _____

_____

_____

_____

When we found out (now or later), I felt… _____

_____

_____

_____

Daddy said… _____

_____

_____

The first baby items we bought you… _____

_____

_____

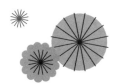
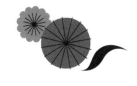

# A Beautiful Sight

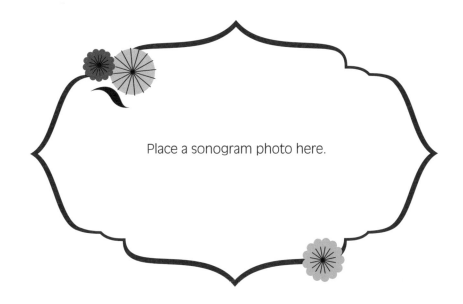

Place a sonogram photo here.

Thoughts: _____

_____

_____

_____

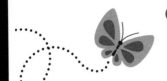 # We're All Aflutter!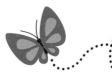

The first time I felt you move was… _____

_____

_____

_____

The sensation feels like… _____

_____

_____

_____

You seem to be most active when… _____

_____

_____

_____

So far I've felt you (check all that apply):

_____ kick                                         _____ hiccup

_____ somersault                               _____ stretch

_____ other: _____

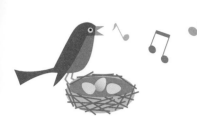 # Sweet Sounds

When I hear these songs, I will think of this special time when I was expecting you… _____

_____

_____

_____

Lately, I like to talk to you about… _____

_____

_____

When Daddy talks to my belly, he says… _____

_____

_____

I like to read these books aloud to you… _____

_____

_____

# Baby Prep

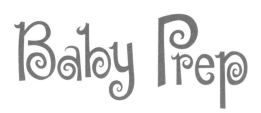

Type of childbirth class: _____

My instructor's name: _____

He/she was… _____

_____

People who went with me… _____

_____

The most surprising thing I learned… _____

_____

_____

I will use these things for my own birth plan… _____

_____

_____

Classmates I befriended… _____

_____

_____

Total number of classes I attended: _____

My tour of the hospital…

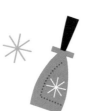
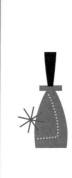

# Mommy Makeover

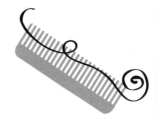

During my pregnancy, my hair has been (check all that apply):

____ shiny and fabulous          ____ out of control          ____ always in a ponytail

____ other: _____

I now walk (check all that apply):

____ with a slight waddle          ____ very slowly          ____ the same as before

____ other: _____

My belly resembles a (check all that apply):

____ small pillow          ____ basketball          ____ large beach ball

____ other: _____

My shoes are (check all that apply):

____ way too small          ____ anything that will stretch          ____ only flip-flops

____ other: _____

Other new physical changes… _____

_____

_____

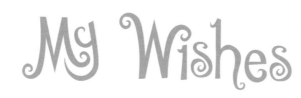 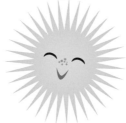

# My Wishes

**I hope that…**

you will inherit these traits from me… _____

_____

_____

and these traits from your father… _____

_____

_____

these are some qualities you don't inherit… _____

_____

_____

I embody the virtues of these amazing mothers… _____

_____

_____

I'll be a good mother because… _____

_____

_____

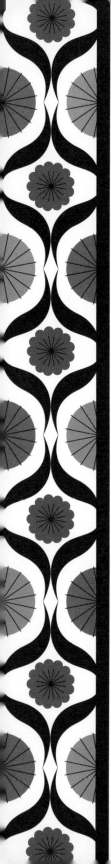

# Summing It Up

**During the second trimester...**

My emotions have been... _____

_____

_____

_____

My symptoms (the good, the bad, and the moody)... _____

_____

_____

_____

Some other noteworthy events... _____

_____

_____

_____

Date _____

**Reflections on my second trimester...**

_____

_____

_____

_____

_____

_____

_____

_____

_____

_____

_____

_____

_____

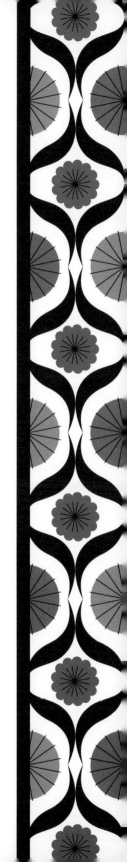

Date _____

# The Third Trimester

What I'm looking forward to... _____

_____

_____

_____

_____

_____

_____

_____

Things I'm going to miss... _____

_____

_____

_____

_____

_____

# Snapshot

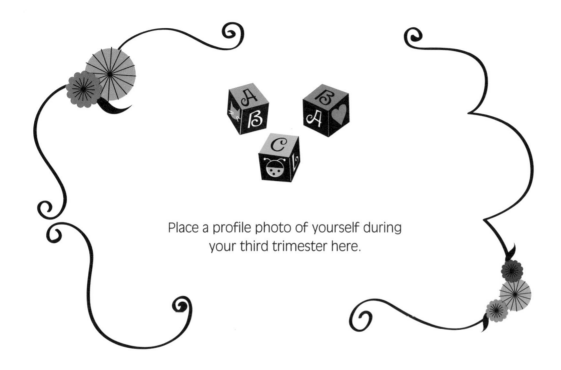

Place a profile photo of yourself during your third trimester here.

Thoughts: _____

_____

_____

_____

_____

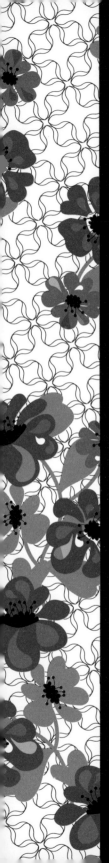

# Nursery Nesting

We started the nursery preparations… _____

_____

_____

The room used to be… _____

_____

We chose this color scheme/overall theme… _____

_____

_____

For furniture and bedding, we liked… _____

_____

_____

The project that gave us the biggest headache… _____

_____

My absolute favorite thing about the nursery… _____

_____

# Nursery Checklist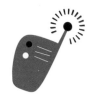

| | On My Registry | Received as Gift | Need to Purchase |
|---|:---:|:---:|:---:|
| Bassinet/crib | ● | ● | ● |
| Mattress/mattress pad | ● | ● | ● |
| Bedding and sheets | ● | ● | ● |
| Changing table | ● | ● | ● |
| Diaper supplies | ● | ● | ● |
| Dresser | ● | ● | ● |
| Bookshelf | ● | ● | ● |
| Baby tub | ● | ● | ● |
| Rocking chair/glider | ● | ● | ● |
| Baby swing | ● | ● | ● |
| Bouncy seat | ● | ● | ● |
| Baby monitor | ● | ● | ● |
| Smoke & carbon monoxide detector | ● | ● | ● |
| Electric outlet covers | ● | ● | ● |
| Storage baskets/bins/bags | ● | ● | ● |
| Closet organizers | ● | ● | ● |
| Portable stereo/sleep sound machine | ● | ● | ● |
| Baby mobile | ● | ● | ● |
| Other(s): | ● | ● | ● |
| | ● | ● | ● |
| | ● | ● | ● |
| | ● | ● | ● |
| | ● | ● | ● |
| | ● | ● | ● |

Use this checklist to get started on your nursery. Talk to family, friends, and experienced moms for more suggestions. For baby's checklist, see page 45.

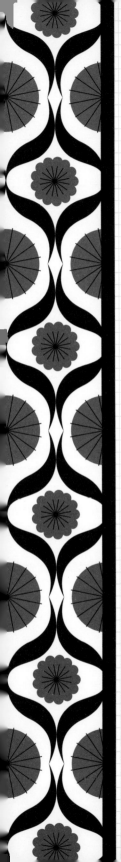

# Map It Out!

Use this page to help design your baby's nursery. You can use the grid to plan the room's layout, or simply paste room ideas from your favorite magazines.

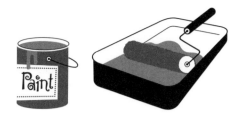

# Picture Perfect

Attach pictures of the nursery before and after it's completed.

**Before**

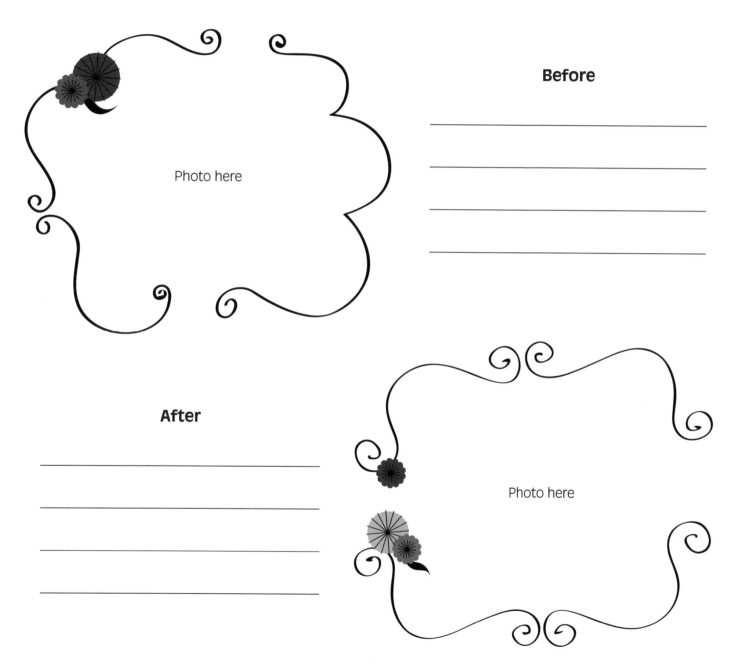

Photo here

_____

_____

_____

_____

**After**

_____

_____

_____

_____

Photo here

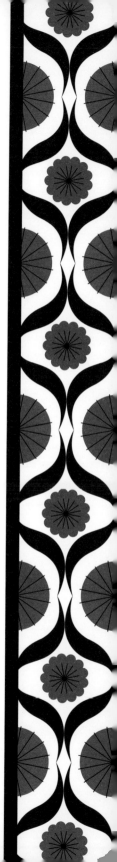

 # Baby Logbook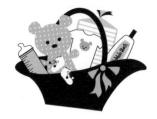

We registered at these stores… _____

_____

_____

The registering process was… _____

_____

_____

A funny moment… _____

*New Kid in Town*

_____

_____

_____

A sweet moment… _____

_____

_____

_____

I got great suggestions from… _____

_____

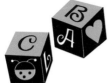 # Baby Checklist

| | On My Registry | Received as Gift | Need to Purchase |
|---|---|---|---|
| Baby carrier | ● | ● | ● |
| Car seat(s) | ● | ● | ● |
| Stroller(s) | ● | ● | ● |
| Diaper bag(s) | ● | ● | ● |
| Swaddling blankets | ● | ● | ● |
| Towels & washcloths | ● | ● | ● |
| Bottles/bottle brushes | ● | ● | ● |
| Breast pump | ● | ● | ● |
| Sleepers | ● | ● | ● |
| Bibs | ● | ● | ● |
| Baby hairbrush/comb | ● | ● | ● |
| Bath products | ● | ● | ● |
| Baby detergent | ● | ● | ● |
| Dishwasher tray (for bottles) | ● | ● | ● |
| Nail clippers | ● | ● | ● |
| Nasal cleaner | ● | ● | ● |
| Teething rings | ● | ● | ● |
| Thermometer | ● | ● | ● |
| Pacifiers | ● | ● | ● |
| Other(s): | ● | ● | ● |
| | ● | ● | ● |
| | ● | ● | ● |
| | ● | | ● |
| | ● | | ● |

Use this checklist to get started on your baby preparations. Talk to family, friends, and experienced moms for more suggestions. For nursery checklist, see page 41.

# The Guessing Game

Fill out the chart below based on family and friends' baby predictions.

| Guesser | Birth Date | Sex and Weight |
|---------|-----------|----------------|
| _____ | _____ | _____ |
| _____ | _____ | _____ |
| _____ | _____ | _____ |
| _____ | _____ | _____ |
| _____ | _____ | _____ |
| _____ | _____ | _____ |
| _____ | _____ | _____ |
| _____ | _____ | _____ |
| _____ | _____ | _____ |
| _____ | _____ | _____ |

Who guessed right!

_____

# Naming You

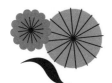
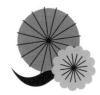

Names we are considering...

Boy Names:                              Girl Names:

_____              _____

_____              _____

_____              _____

_____              _____

_____              _____

_____              _____

_____              _____

Reasons why... _____

_____

_____

_____

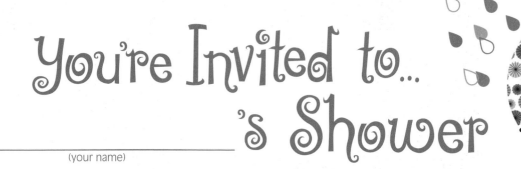

# You're Invited to...
# _____'s Shower
(your name)

Date & Time: _____

Hosted by: _____

Theme: _____

Friends and family who attended... _____

_____

_____

_____

Some wonderful gifts... _____

_____

_____

_____

What I will remember most... _____

_____

_____

# Bring this book to your shower, and ask guests to write their well-wishes for baby.

Guest: _____

Wishes: _____

_____

Guest: _____

Wishes: _____

_____

Guest: _____

Wishes: _____

_____

Guest: _____

Wishes: _____

_____

Guest: _____

Wishes: _____

_____

Guest: _____

Wishes: _____

_____

Guest: _____

Wishes: _____

_____

Guest: _____

Wishes: _____

_____

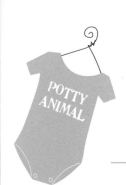

# You're Invited to...

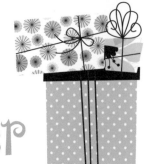

_____ 's Shower

(your name)

Date & Time: _____

Hosted by: _____

Theme: _____

Friends and family who attended... _____

_____

_____

_____

Some wonderful gifts... _____

_____

_____

What I will remember most... _____

_____

_____

Use these pages for any additional showers you may have.

Bring this book to your shower, and ask guests
to write their well-wishes for baby.

Guest: _____
Wishes: _____
_____

Guest: _____
Wishes: _____
_____

Guest: _____
Wishes:_____
_____

Guest: _____
Wishes: _____
_____

Guest: _____
Wishes: _____
_____

Guest: _____
Wishes: _____
_____

Guest: _____
Wishes: _____
_____

Guest: _____
Wishes: _____
_____

# Shower Mementos

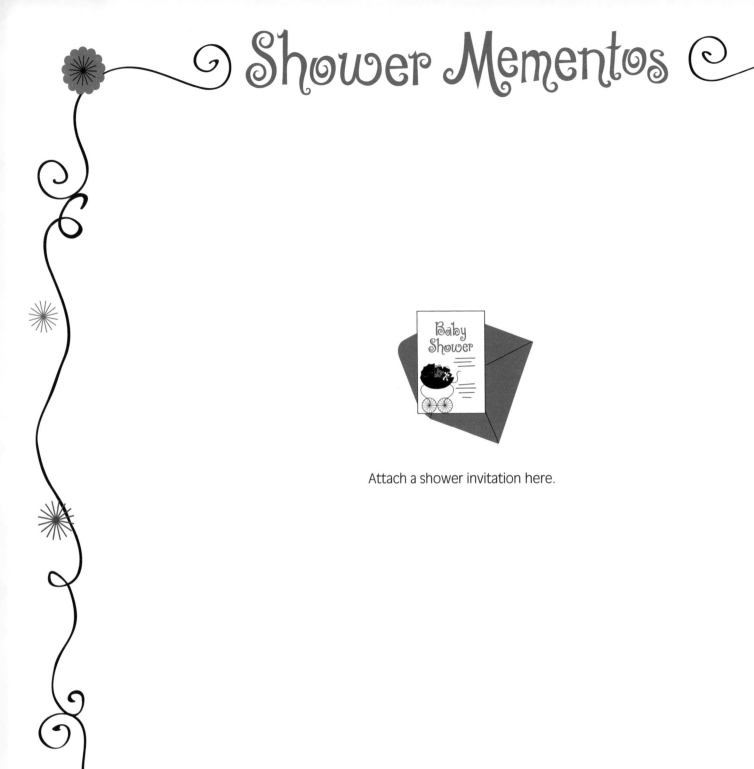

Attach a shower invitation here.

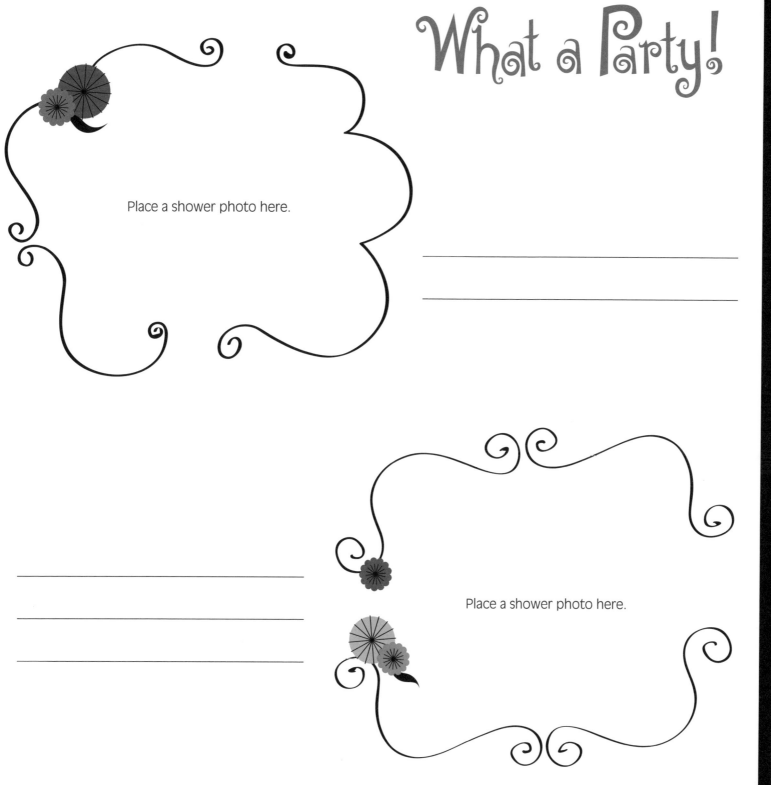

# What a Party!

Place a shower photo here.

Place a shower photo here.

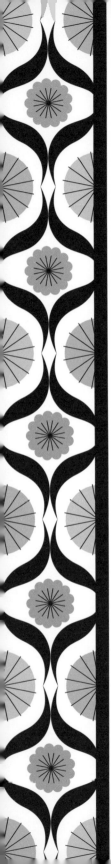

# Some Friendly Advice

People I've talked to for advice during my pregnancy... _____

_____

_____

_____

_____

I've needed the most help with... _____

_____

_____

_____

Advice that's helped me... _____

_____

_____

_____

_____

Some funny suggestions I've received… _____

_____

_____

_____

_____

And some terrible ones… _____

_____

_____

_____

_____

_____

At this point in my pregnancy, I feel comfortable with… _____

_____

_____

_____

_____

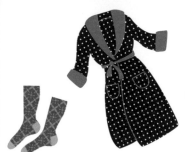

# Packing Checklist

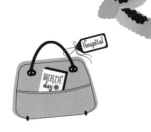

| For Me: | I'll Pack It | Dad's Packing It | Double Duty |
|---|:---:|:---:|:---:|
| Toiletries | ● | ● | ● |
| Robe | ● | ● | ● |
| Pajamas/lounge wear | ● | ● | ● |
| Slippers | ● | ● | ● |
| Socks | ● | ● | ● |
| Nursing bra/pads | ● | ● | ● |
| Maternity underwear | ● | ● | ● |
| Change of clothes | ● | ● | ● |
| Extra pillow | ● | ● | ● |
| Phone/camera | ● | ● | ● |
| Chargers | ● | ● | ● |
| Music | ● | ● | ● |
| Hospital paperwork | ● | ● | ● |
| This book | ● | ● | ● |
| Other(s): | ● | ● | ● |
|  | ● | ● | ● |
|  | ● | ● | ● |
|  | ● | ● | ● |

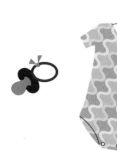 # Packing Checklist

| For Baby: | I'll Pack It | Dad's Packing It | Double Duty |
|---|---|---|---|
| Car seat | ● | ● | ● |
| Blankets | ● | ● | ● |
| Diaper bag | ● | ● | ● |
| Diapers | ● | ● | ● |
| Onesies | ● | ● | ● |
| Sleepers | ● | ● | ● |
| Pacifiers | ● | ● | ● |
| Baby hat | ● | ● | ● |
| Socks/booties | ● | ● | ● |
| Going-home outfit | ● | ● | ● |
| Other(s): | ● | ● | ● |
| | ● | ● | ● |
| | ● | ● | ● |
| | ● | ● | ● |
| | ● | ● | ● |
| | ● | ● | ● |
| | ● | ● | ● |

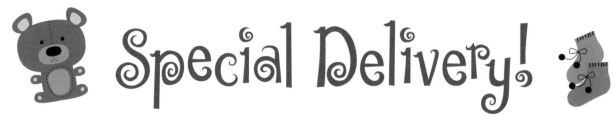

# Special Delivery!

I knew it was time when… _____

_____

_____

_____

_____

The ride to the hospital was… _____

_____

_____

_____

_____

My labor was… _____

_____

_____

_____

You were delivered by… _____

_____

Who was in the room to greet you... _____

_____

_____

_____

And who came to see you during our hospital stay... _____

_____

_____

_____

Everyone thinks you look like... _____

_____

_____

_____

Plans for the trip home... _____

_____

_____

_____

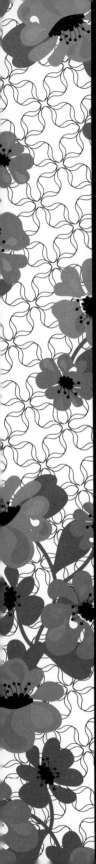

# It's Official!

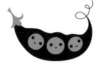

Place a picture of your
newborn baby here.

Full name: _____

Place of birth: _____

Delivered by: _____

Date of birth: _____ Time of birth:_____

Weight: _____ Length: _____

Eye color: _____ Hair color: _____

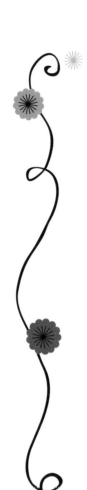
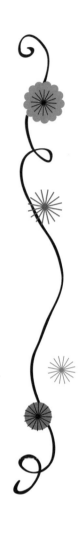

# Baby of Mine

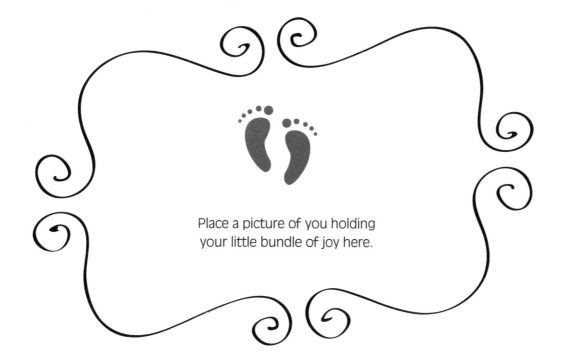

Place a picture of you holding
your little bundle of joy here.

Thoughts: _____

_____

_____

_____

_____

Date _____

When I first held you... _____

_____

_____

_____

_____

_____

_____

_____

_____

_____

_____

_____

_____

_____

**Ask Daddy or a loved one to journal about the day baby was born.**

_____ thought ... _____
(name)

_____

_____

_____

_____

_____

_____

_____

_____

_____

_____

_____

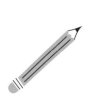
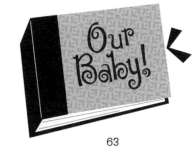

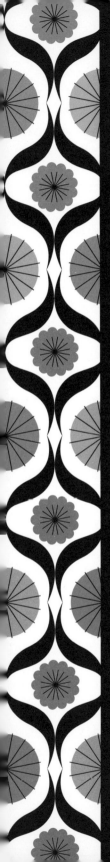

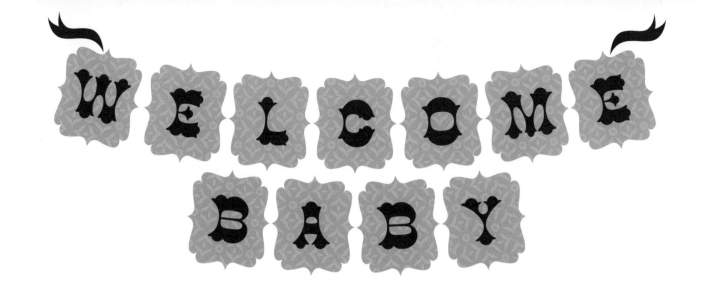

WELCOME BABY

Attach baby's birth announcement here.

Thoughts: _____

_____

_____

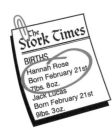

# Read All About It!

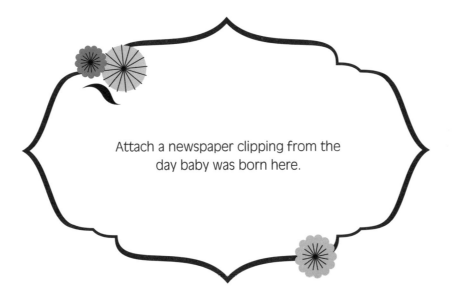

Attach a newspaper clipping from the day baby was born here.

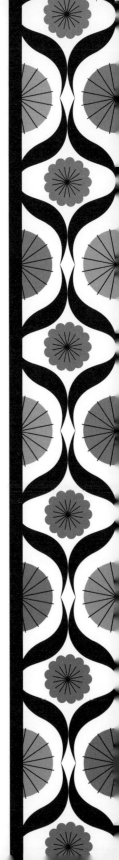

Thoughts: _____

_____

_____

# Our New Family

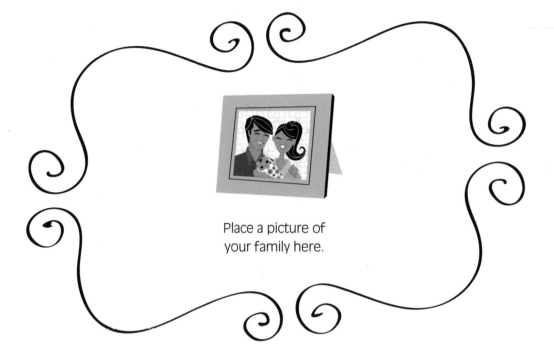

Place a picture of
your family here.

Thoughts: _____

_____

_____

_____

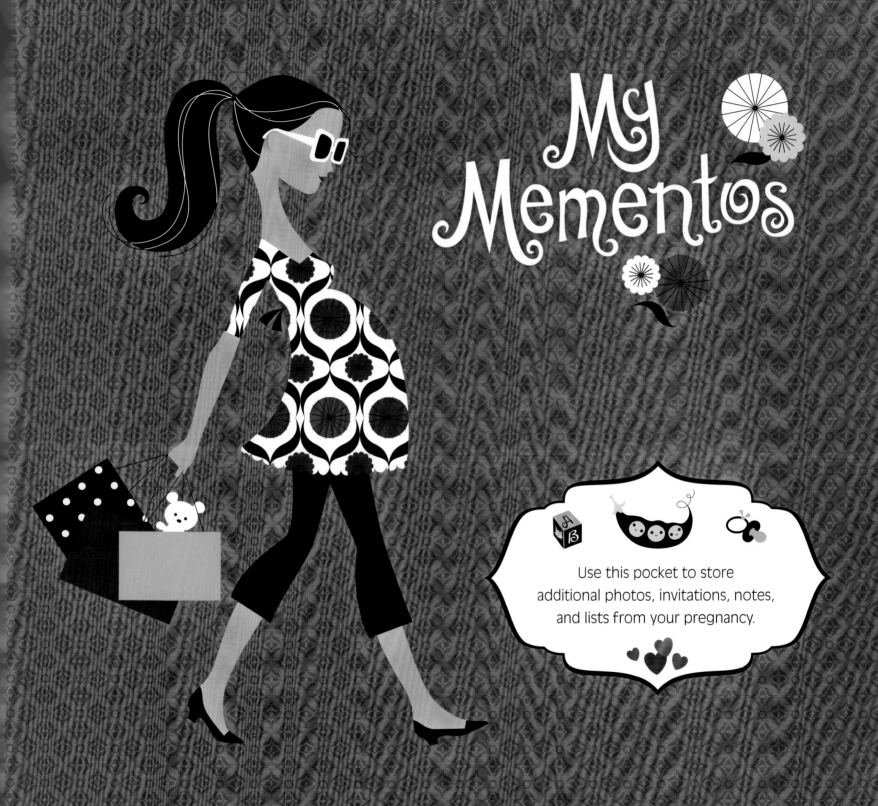

My Mementos

Use this pocket to store
additional photos, invitations, notes,
and lists from your pregnancy.